Introduction

Swinging is a lifestyle choice that is becoming more and more popular these days. Before we made our first venture into what is known as "the lifestyle", we read a few books and magazine

articles to try and prepare us for what lied ahead. The majority of the books all told us how exciting it is, how it enhances your sex life, and how fun it can be.

While a lot of that is true, one thing a lot of the books failed to mention are some of the negative aspects and pitfalls of swinging. I am not a professional writer by any means, but my goal is to help as many couples as possible make an informed decision before exploring the world of swinging. Sit back, keep an open mind, and enjoy.

Andre Keith

Chapter 1

<u>What is Swinging?</u>

Swinging is often known as partner swapping, partner sharing, or wife swapping in some media circles. A lot of people have the misconception that swinging is a new phenomenon, but swinging (also referred to as "the lifestyle") has been around for centuries. In ancient times, most rulers had wives as well as concubines. There are multiple references to concubines in the Bible, in Judaism, and in the Muslim world.

Ancient Greece and Rome are both well known for throwing lavish parties for the purposes of sexual pleasure which would include voyeurism, threesomes, and orgies. Group sex and orgies are commonly depicted in ancient Greek and Roman drawings. Benjamin Franklin was known to be a nudist and a swinger. Marie Antoinette of France was also rumored to throw orgies during her time.

Modern day swinging supposedly owes its origin to US Air Force pilots back during WWII. Folklore tells us that a close comradery arose between pilots during this time, and pilots were called upon to "take care" of each other's wives both sexually and emotionally if something happened to the husband. Other urban legends point to the origin of modern day swinging to Air Force pilots and their wives who were stationed in California. In 1963, the Sexual Freedom League was formed, which was a precursor to what is now the North American Swing Club Association (NASCA – www.nasca.com). The purpose of this organization is to make sure that people have accurate information about swinging, since swingers were often portrayed in a negative light by the media.

You might have also heard of there being "key parties" during this time. A key party was a party held at someone's house where all of the husbands tossed their car/house keys into a basket. The wives would then close their eyes, reach into the basket and pick out a set of keys. Whoever the keys belonged to was her sexual partner for the evening.

The 1970's are often referred to as "The Swinging 70's" as swinging started to become more mainstream and prevalent. Swinging really began to take off during the 1990's when the internet made it easier for couples in the lifestyle to find each other. Today there are numerous websites, international vacation resorts, and night clubs all over the world solely devoted to people who are interested in the swinging lifestyle.

I know you're probably surprised at how short this chapter is on the history of swinging, but I personally hate reading books where the author just puts meaningless words on a page only for the purpose of making the book longer. There's plenty of websites you can visit if you would like to know more about the history of swinging.

Types of Swinging

This list is by no means exhaustive, but here are some of the more common types of swinging.

Voyeurism

One of the dictionaries I have describes voyeurism as the compulsion to seek sexual gratification by secretly looking at sexual objects or acts; such as the actions of Peeping Tom. I don't quite agree with this definition because the term "Peeping Tom" has a negative connotation that makes voyeurism seem as if it's something un-natural.

Voyeurism for most people is a natural gateway into the world of swinging. Those just dipping their toes into the lifestyle pool for the first time often start out as voyeurs. Voyeurs love to watch others engage in sex, and sometimes enjoy being watched themselves.

Soft Swapping

This usually involves two couples getting together sexually, however no one exchanges partners. Usually the two females will start off having sex with each other first, and each male participates only with his own partner. A lot of couples that are new to swinging usually start out this way, as they aren't quite prepared to watch their partner have sex with someone of the opposite sex. For some, soft swap can also include other non-penetrating activities such as oral sex, rimming, (licking around the anus) and passionate kissing.

This type of fun usually takes place in the same room, but can also happen in separate rooms.

Full Swapping

Full swapping consists of two or more couples getting together, and each male has sex with the other person's spouse or partner. It may also involve the females engaging in sex with each other as well.

Cuckold

By definition, a cuckold is the husband of a cheating wife or partner. In this category, it usually refers to a man who enjoys his woman having sex with other males. Often times the man will invite another male (also known or referred to as a "bull") over to have sex with his wife while he watches. Other men sometimes just enjoy the mental aspect of knowing his wife had sex with another guy while he was at work. This can lead to an aggressive session of lovemaking when he comes home, to "punish" her for being bad.

There may also be some form of humiliation involved for the guy who is watching, such as having to get drinks for his wife and her lover, or "clean up" after sex. I've seen a few videos where the women will insult her husband during the sex, saying things like "You wish you could fuck me this good, don't you?" or "This is HIS pussy now, not yours."

Lately at sex stores I've seen cuckold cock cages. These cages are meant to go over a man's penis, almost like a chastity device. Some men derive intense satisfaction knowing they are restrained while watching their woman have sex with another guy. While some believe it's just "condoned" infidelity, for a lot of couples it adds excitement to their sex lives without the feelings of betrayal that come with cheating.

Threesomes

A threesome is a group of three people engaging in sexual activity together. Usually this consists of a couple inviting a male or female over for a night of fun. The most common threesome involves two women and one male, often referred to as a FMF threesome. Lots of couples also engage in MFM threesomes so a woman can experience being with two males at the same time. MFM threesomes are also a good way for bisexual males to have the best of both worlds.

BDSM

BDSM is an acronym for Bondage & Discipline, Domination & Submission, and Sadism & Masochism. Some people have their own interpretation for the acronym, but this is what we'll use for the purpose of this book. BDSM can be described as a type of role play or lifestyle choice between two or more individuals who use their experiences of pain and power to create sexual tension, pleasure, and release. This can also apply to people who like to be tied up or spanked during sex. Some even take it to the extreme where a male of the relationship is called the Daddy or Master, and the female is the Submissive or Slave. Roles can also be reversed as there are plenty of Female Masters as well.

There was one evening where we visited a swinger-friendly hotel bar in our area to celebrate a couples anniversary. Everyone who was invited was a swinger, so there was lots of kissing, hugging and groping going on. This one female was talking to me for a while, and then I didn't see her again for a few hours. I was informed that her Master hadn't given her permission to speak to guys that night, and he took her back to their hotel room to "punish" her. Her punishment consisted of getting spanked, and then having sex. When she came back to the bar she had quite the Cheshire grin on her face.

BDSM really isn't a swinging type per se, however it does seem to be something that a lot of swingers enjoy.

Gangbangs

A gangbang is a group session where several people have sex with one person in particular, usually all at the same time, or one person after another. This is seen in porn a lot where one female may be having sex with three or four guys at the same time. Participants of a gang bang can engage in anal, vaginal, oral sex, or even double penetration.

Chapter 2

Why Do People Swing?

Some people will wonder why do couples participate in swinging?
Why would someone want to let another person have sex with their
spouse or partner? I asked myself this same question when my
wife and I first got married. She had previously been a part of the
lifestyle with another partner before she and I even met. I thought
to myself that there was no way in hell I would ever enjoy watching
my wife have sex with another male. It was never, EVER going to
happen. The ironic thing about this statement is that we got
married at a clothing-optional resort.

My thinking back then was, "Well sure I like watching naked people,
but no way are we swinging." Even then at that resort, the seeds of
swinging had been planted. The resort had a rooftop Jacuzzi that
was the size of a normal swimming pool. All around the Jacuzzis
there were cabana beds with fire pits.

At night time, there was something very sensual watching naked
bodies of all shapes and sizes relax in the Jacuzzi or on the beds.

Our first trip into voyeurism started here, as we watched some of the couples have sex on the beds. The highlight of our trip at this resort was having sex on one of the beds on a particular night, while there was a couple right beside us in another bed. It was a major turn-on watching them have sex, and knowing they were watching us as well.

Fast forward a year and we visited our first swingers club to watch other couples have sex. Later that same year we visited Hedonism II for an anniversary trip, and the rest is history. What changed my mind? Well here are a few good reasons why couples start swinging.

It Is Exciting

This is probably the number one benefit and reason people will give for swinging. Having sex with other people with your partner's permission can be extremely exciting. It's really the best of both worlds. You get all of the love, closeness, and sex from a "traditional" relationship, but you also get to enjoy sex with other people you are attracted to. It's also an erotic rush visiting sex clubs, or looking online at swinger websites to check out who you want to hook up with.

When you find another person or couple that you are sexually compatible with and attracted to, you feel like you've hit the jackpot. There are also all kinds of fun, adults-only resorts you can visit that cater to nudists and swingers in great locations like Jamaica, Mexico, and the Dominican Republic.

The great thing about clothing-optional resorts is you don't have to pack nearly as many clothes, which makes for a more enjoyable travelling experience in my opinion. Also, who wants to listen to other people's kids running around all over the place when they're on vacation? Not me, I'll pick an adults-only resort any day of the week over visiting a place with a bunch of kids. They even have clothing-optional cruises now, which always sell out almost as fast as they are announced.

Threesomes are Awesome

Let me repeat. Threesomes are not just awesome, they are INSANELY awesome. As for me, the only thing that's better than having two women pleasing you at the same time is having THREE women pleasing you. For women, having a threesome is fantastic because it allows you to be adored and ravaged by two males (or a man and woman) at the same time.

Some women also have fantasies of double-penetration (one penis in the vagina, one in the anus) and derive incredible orgasms from having their G-spot hit from both sides. Since some women are capable of having multiple orgasms, threesomes are a fantastic way for her to be truly satisfied as most women have more sexual stamina than a typical male. A number of women have fantasies of being with another female, so threesomes are a perfect way to make that fantasy a reality.

If you've never had a threesome before, I highly recommend you put it on your bucket list. For you guys out there, you know how awesome it is to have your woman riding you? Well imagine another woman sitting on your face making out with your woman while she rides you. Told you it was awesome.

All of Your Fantasies Fulfilled

As I've alluded to before, swinging is one the best ways to get all of your fantasies fulfilled. Do you fantasize about giving your husband a threesome? You can make that happen. Do you fantasize about watching people have sex? Watching people have sex on TV doesn't do it justice. You can visit a local swingers club and make that happen.

Watching live sex is way more erotic and sensual than watching it on TV. During the course of swinging, you'll probably discover even more fantasies that you never realized you had before, and you can make most of them come true.

You Will Make Some New Friends

One of the BEST things about swinging is you start meeting more open-minded people. When we visited our first clothing-optional resort for our wedding, my wife was fearful that we would be hit on all day by people wanting to have sex with us. This was the furthest thing from the truth. All the people we met were super nice, very laid back with no pressure at all. One of the couples was even nice enough to attend our wedding ceremony on the beach (clothed) and we met some awesome people.

Not to say that your regular friends aren't great, but let's be honest here. When you're around other "normal" (often referred to as "vanilla") couples at a party, most of the conversation centers around work and kids. When you're around other swinger couples they may still be talking about work, but conversations usually gravitate around sex, and you get to hear what exciting sexual escapades they've had recently. They can also refer you to other swingers that you may be compatible with.

Also, having swinger friends makes for a very interesting birthday party. If you're a male and it's your birthday, it's not uncommon for the women to "fixate" on the birthday boy while all the other males cheer him on. I don't know about you, but I'd much rather be wished happy birthday with multiple pairs of breasts in my face than have Pete from accounting blab away about how smart his kid is, or the new route he found to work.

For my wife's birthday one year, it was her idea to invite over a single female and a single male for some sexual fun. That night ended up with me and the woman having anal sex, while my wife and the male were having anal sex at the same time. Talk about a memorable birthday.

It's An Incredible Ego Boost

It's very flattering to know that somebody else wants to screw your brains out. It's an even bigger ego boost if they want to keep hooking up with you because you're awesome in bed. If you're a stereotypical "nice guy" like myself, we're always second guessing ourselves when it comes to wondering if someone is attracted to us or not. In the swinging lifestyle, you instantly know who is attracted to you.

Being in the lifestyle is every empowering for women, and the women are usually a little more aggressive when they are swinging. It's not uncommon for a woman to approach a man and express sexual interest right away. Often times when you go to hug a woman, you may get what's called a "lifestyle hug" where she pulls you in close and squeezes your butt during the hug. This is awesome for guys who aren't used to women approaching them.

Women in the lifestyle don't have to be worried about being labeled by society for being sexually forward.

Sometimes when you settle down with someone, you forget just how attractive you or your partner are. It's easy to forget that your woman is a sex goddess that other men salivate over. Swinging can potentially open up a whole new door of appreciation for your partner, and she can also be turned on knowing other women desire you. I know this will sound sexist, but nothing in my opinion will inspire more sex from your woman than her seeing how much other women desire you.

You'll Learn Some New Sexual Tricks

Everyone has different sexual tricks they've mastered over the years, so it's always a great thing when you discover something new. One of the things we learned is that my wife can squirt (female ejaculation) during anal sex. Neither of us knew this before, so this was an awesome discovery. I have also learned how to make my wife and other women squirt by using my hands, and it works almost 100% of the time. Awesome.

Since you two are discovering new things about each other and getting to experience new people, your sex life will never get boring and dull. Variety is the spice of life.

Your Woman is Naughtier Than You Ever Imagined

Chris Rock is right. During one of his stand-up performances, he proclaims "Your woman is nastier than you ever imagined." He is absolutely right.

I vividly remember my night of enlightenment. Back in my single days, there was this one woman that used to be a booty call. This woman was a card-carrying feminist. There was all types of feminist propaganda in her apartment, and any conversation with her always included a speech about how women are treated unfairly in society. Of course I would usually nod my head in agreement with whatever she was saying, since I didn't want to mess up my chances of getting laid by upsetting her.

One night I visited her and I was upset about something. I don't even remember what it was that upset me, but I wasn't in the mood to hear any speech about how males are responsible for the downfall of humanity. I also started thinking about the few weeks we'd been messing around, and she hadn't given me a blowjob yet but I'd gone down on her plenty of times. She started in with her usual conversation, and I just stopped her dead in her tracks. I grabbed her by the hand and took her to the bedroom. I noticed a handkerchief on her dresser and I used that to blindfold her. I put my penis right on her lips and she eagerly gave me a blowjob. Interestingly enough, if I would've politely asked I probably would've gotten a pretty lame blowjob, if one at all.

That night when we were having sex, I didn't treat her as some delicate creature like I always had, because I didn't care about getting kicked out of the bed. While we were having sex, I leaned over and told her she was going to be my sex slave and do whatever I said. I also smacked her on the ass, which I had never done before because she said it objectified women. Now I just KNEW in my mind, that this feminist woman would sit straight up in bed and object to me thinking she was going to submit to me sexually.

Did this happen? Absolutely not. As a matter of fact, that brought about the biggest orgasm I had ever been able to give her before. I would have never expected this woman to respond the way she did, but it was an eye-opening experience for me. It's amazing the sexual things people can do in the heat of the moment.

I also used to have this female friend that would complain about her husband being too gentle with her. She said (and this is word for word) "I tell him to go harder and he just says I'm his little princess, and he can't treat me that way. I wish for once he would just put me in a corner, bend me over and fuck me in my ass." The point I'm trying to make here is that your woman is more open to doing things than you think.

That's right, your sweet little sugar plum, princess, sweet cakes, or whatever name you have for your woman WANTS you to corrupt her. Don't believe me? Next time you're in line at the grocery store, take a glance at the Cosmo magazine cover. I'd be willing to bet one of the articles featured is something about "how to drive a man wild in bed" or something like that.

Are you tired of the same old boring sex and the same lazy blowjob you've been getting for years? Well guess what, your woman is tired of it too. Swinging can help spice things up a little. When I first watched my wife giving a blowjob to another man, I honestly was amazed at the energy and effort she put into it. I found that after we started swinging, I started getting those same, energetic blowjobs that I used to get when we first started dating.

Let's be honest guys, when you go down on your woman you probably don't do it with the same enthusiasm you used to when you first started dating, so it works both ways. Swinging can definitely draw out your woman's naughty side in ways you never imagined.

Chapter 3

Downside of Swinging

I know that I've made swinging out to be the greatest thing since sliced bread, and it certainly can be. There are numerous reasons and benefits of swinging, but it would be irresponsible of me if I didn't mention some of the negative aspects of it as well.

If You Have Problems in Your Relationship, They Will Become Worse

Swinging is absolutely NOT a cure all for your relationship. If you have major problems in your relationship, swinging will highlight those problems and make them worse. For those of you with lots of relationship problems, you should avoid swinging all together. If you have a jealous personality, are insecure, and don't spend enough time together already, swinging will bring these problems to the spotlight.

If you are truly not in love or have any other major issues, swinging will make things much worse. I remember one time we invited this couple over for some fun with us and another single guy. Well this couple was obviously having some problems, and it started to become clear that they weren't on the same page at all. They actually started arguing in front of us. Talk about awkward.

STD's

Although most swingers are very strict about using condoms, that doesn't mean you're going to be immune from catching an STD. Most of us don't use condoms or dental dams when engaging in oral sex, so you can still catch something. One of the DUMBEST things we ever did was choose to go bareback (no condoms) with one of the couples we played with. Of course they assured us we were the only people they went bareback with, but how did we really know they were being truthful?

Finally I came to my senses and told them that we need to go back to using condoms. A few weeks later, I saw a picture on a swinging website of them having a threesome with a female, and the male was having anal sex with that female and wasn't wearing a condom. Never feel like you are offending someone by making sure condoms are always used. I've seen a few swinging profiles online where couples have caught herpes from other couples who weren't honest about having an STD. Protect yourselves at all times.

Your Woman Will Get More Action Than You

This is something that couples rarely think about when they start swinging, but it's something that really needs to be considered. There are WAY more available guys in the swinger world than there are single females. When I say more, I literally mean 2 to 3 times more guys available. As a matter of fact, single females in the swinger world are referred to as "unicorns", and for good reason. It will take you a day at the most to find a single male to give your wife a threesome, but it took us almost an entire year for us to find a female for a threesome.

If you think females are flaky on normal dating websites, it's only worse when swinging; they are literally three times as flaky when you're looking on swinging websites. There have been plenty of times where we have a meeting or dinner date set up with a single female, only to have her cancel at the last minute with an incredulous reason. Some of the online profiles of single women are also completely fake.

When you attend a swingers party or club, your wife will have PLENTY of guys to choose from and hook up with, while you may only have one or two prospects. This can lead to a lot of frustration, and even resentment if you don't know this before you get started. Trust me, I know from personal experience.

There Are Lots of People Better-Looking Than You

To piggyback on the previous topic, not only are there 2 to 3 times the amount of guys, there will be plenty of guys who are in better shape than you are, handsome, and lots will have bigger dicks. Sometimes it's not easy watching your woman have sex with a guy who's taller, in better shape, and is hung like he should be on a porno movie set. This can be especially difficult when you may not have many options available to you because of the scarcity of women.

To compound the issue, most of the women you get to have sex will NOT look better than your wife. I'm not trying to insult anyone here, I'm just being honest. Most of the women you get to have sex with will be on the same level of attractiveness as your wife or below.

On the off chance you do get to have sex with someone who is incredibly sexy, your wife/girlfriend may have her own issues with this. It also may not be easy for your wife to watch you moan in ecstasy as a beautiful woman pleases you.

Cheating

You would think that cheating wouldn't occur when people are swinging. You're thinking that you get the best of both worlds. You still get to have sex with your partner, plus you get to have sex with other people. Why mess that up with cheating? It seems highly illogical to cheat when you're already getting to enjoy being with other people. See that's your logical mind coming into play, and we all know that logic doesn't work too well when raw emotions are involved.

Most people have the assumption that single females are the biggest threat to a relationship while swinging, but surprisingly single males are usually the worst offenders. Single males get a bad rap in the swinging world, and to be honest it's for good reason. Shockingly enough, quite often it is the female half of a relationship that ends up cheating. Yes of course there are males who cheat in this scenario as well, but usually not since they think they're already getting the best of both worlds.

Single guys can be the worst offenders because of the scarcity of females. Since most couples are looking for other couples or single females, this leaves single guys with even fewer options. Once a single guy finds a willing couple, he just might put the full court press onto your girlfriend/spouse.   He'll start telling her things like "If you were my woman, I'd never share you". Every male half of a swinging couple who is reading this right now is nodding their head in agreement as they've dealt with this first hand, or have witnessed this themselves. Sometimes your partner may start to get emotionally attached to someone they like having sex with, and the rest is history.

Single females on the other hand usually have so many male suitors and couples pursuing them that they normally don't have the time to fixate on someone's husband/boyfriend. One single female told us that the first week she signed up for a profile on a swinging website, she literally had over 200 emails. This may seem like a very high number, but really it boils down to supply and demand. There are way too many couples and single males trying to get the attention of only a handful of women.

I know, I get it. YOUR woman will never cheat on you in a million years. Here's something you need to understand. EVERYONE is capable of cheating and no relationship is completely immune to it. Let that sink in for a moment.

ALL PEOPLE ARE CAPABLE OF CHEATING.

Whether your partner does it or not is another story. The website Ashley Madison (a website for married adulterers) reports that on the day after Mother's Day, they see an increase of over 400% from the usual number of women who sign up on any given day. That's right, over 400% in case you wondering if I added an extra zero by mistake. Sometimes all it takes is the right opportunity and situation for it to happen. I can speak to this first hand as it happened in my relationship, and I never thought in a million years my wife would cheat on me while we were swinging. Neither did she for that matter, and we almost ended up in a bitter divorce over it. I know of this happening to other couples as well. Also be aware that cheating isn't just physical, it can be mental. I can admit that I also started to develop an emotional connection with one of the females I had sex with.

You May Lose Your Connection

This also follows up on the cheating issue. We all know how thrilling it is to get attention from the opposite sex. I found that I was spending an enormous amount of time online searching for new people to have sex with. I also found that my wife started texting me less and less during the work day, while she was busy texting other guys. I was so focused on getting a threesome, that's all I seemed to focus on.

Where we used to normally talk about different things, most of our conversations now revolved around swinging. All of our free time seemed to be spent trying to find new sexual conquests, attending or hosting sex parties, and sexting other people. It got so bad at one point, I remember one night we were both sitting on the couch beside each other, both texting other people.

There's only so much emotional energy people have, and when some of that energy is spent on other people, that leaves less energy and emotion for your relationship. I know of one couple that got divorced after 15 years of marriage because they were having more sex with other people than they were with each other. It's hard enough for a marriage to survive the normal stressors of work and bills, and adding swinging to it can open up a new can of worms.

When I say that my wife and I almost divorced, I literally mean we were a gnat's ass hair away from it happening. She had already got her own individual cellphone line, and already had money saved up to get her own place. That's how close we were to splitting up. Lots of therapy, communication, and a 2 year break from swinging helped to save our marriage.

It's Addictive

Swinging is highly addictive and once you start, it may be almost impossible to stop. My wife and I are living proof of this. It's exciting meeting a new couple for drinks to see if you have a connection. After we tried swinging for the first time, we said we didn't want to do it again. Then a few months later my wife was mentioning it again. Every time we said we were going to take a break from it, we found ourselves getting sucked back into it because we missed all the sexual excitement and attention.

I look back now at the countless hours I spent browsing websites for prospects, and it's honestly a damn shame. I spent hours a day that could have been devoted to finishing my degree, looking for a new job, working out, or just spending time with my wife. I would even be on my cellphone at work browsing the website, constantly looking for new people. Even other couples have told us that they don't think they could ever go back to having a "normal" relationship because they would miss all of the fun. Once Pandora's Box is opened, it's hard to close it back up.

Judgement

There are a lot of seriously negative connotations out there about swingers. We don't love our spouses. We're just doing this as a way to cheat. Swingers are sexual deviants with no morals. Even though we're supposed to be an enlightened society, these attitudes still persist. You can go online as we speak about how some swinger clubs are being shut down because some cities don't want "that type of behavior" going on in their city. We recently opened up a business checking account and one of the rules we had to agree to was "no adult entertainment" businesses allowed.

If you're an active participant in your community, you can pretty much guarantee that you will be ostracized and looked down upon if your neighbors ever find out. One guy I know told some of the other guys at his job about he and his wife being swingers, and they just shook their heads at him. They wonder how in the world can he let his wife have sex with another man, but the irony is that half of these guys cheat on their wives. One of my wife's good male friends said that no male should ever want to see his wife have sex with another man. At first this made me feel really guilty and almost ashamed of being a swinger.

Then I thought about it more. This guy has a really insecure wife, is on his second marriage, and he only gets to have sex with her a few times a month. So who is he to give advice on what works and what doesn't work? One of the well-known swinger clubs in our area once tried to make a sizable donation to a Cancer foundation, but the foundation rejected the money because of who it came from. I wish I was making this up but I'm not. It's a prime example of just how petty and judgmental some people can be towards swinging.

Just know that if other people find out, some of them will look down their noses at you. People who you call friends may no longer want anything to do with you. Always remember though, what works for one relationship doesn't work for all. There is no rulebook out there that says there is only one way to have a successful relationship. People often mean well, but they are just figuring things out as they go along, just like you are. Decide what makes you and your partner happy, and then DO IT. As long as what you are doing isn't causing harm to anybody else.....GO FOR IT.

Too often we let the imaginary rules of society determine what it is that we're supposed to be doing with our lives. Make up your own rules and boundaries, and stop letting other people dictate what will work in YOUR relationship. One of my friends said it best: Being a swinger is like opening up a bag of chips in church. Everybody looks at you in disgust, but deep down inside they want some too.

Chapter 4

Rules to Make Swinging Work

Take Breaks

It is imperative that you take some breaks from time to time from swinging. This is the one thing that couples often forget to do, and it usually leads to big trouble. Breaks are important in my opinion because swinging should not dominate your social life, and in no way should it overtake the connection you have with your partner.

Taking a break allows you to re-establish your connection with each other and give each other undivided attention. After you've been playing for a while, I suggest taking at least a month-long break to focus on just each other.

Your Partner is Your Primary Focus

Swinging is fun and exciting, but never lose focus of the fact that your partner should be the one getting the majority of your attention. Healthy relationships take work and energy to maintain. Don't spend more time and energy trying to find swinging partners than you do on your relationship.

Also, be aware of people who appear to be too needy or always want your attention. Remember you are NOT in this lifestyle to have a new girlfriend or boyfriend, you already have one of those, and it should be made VERY clear to everyone else. Sometimes there are cases where single people start getting emotionally attached and start trying to steal your mate away.

At this one party we attended, a single male actually got mad at my wife because she had sex with someone else first that night. This type of needy behavior is never to be tolerated. There was another single male that felt "hurt" that my wife chose another guy as her first hall pass instead of him. When you encounter these type of people, I suggest cutting them off and no longer dealing with them. These emotionally attached people can cause all sorts of problems with your relationship if you enable the behavior.

Clear, Open, and Honest Communication

If you follow no other rule, this is the main one to follow. You MUST be able to communicate with one another about what you are feeling, along with your likes and dislikes. If something happens during the course of swinging that you don't like (and it will, trust me) then speak up and tell your partner. If your partner did something that upset you, don't come at them in an accusatory manner because that will just make them defensive. Make a promise to each other that no matter what happens while swinging, that you will talk about it afterwards in a calm and rational manner.

One of the biggest mistakes we made when we first started swinging was the lack of open communication. There were times where she wanted to stop swinging, but didn't say anything because she thought I would be unhappy. At other times, I didn't want to share her anymore but I didn't want to ruin all of the fun she was having. It's important that you communicate and respect each other's feelings.

You also need to define rules for what is and isn't okay right from the beginning. Don't just assume that doing something is okay, you should talk about it first. Is it okay to allow for passionate kissing? Is anal sex okay? Is it okay to swallow if a guy cums during a blowjob? Is hugging after sex okay? Is it okay to give someone else a threesome? These are things you need to talk about and discuss beforehand.

A great way of doing this is after you've been to a party, or have had people over, lay in bed with each other and have an honest discussion about how things went. It's important to feel like you can be honest and forthcoming without the other getting mad. Learn to confide in each other, not other people. Once you start confiding in others (other than a therapist) about the things you don't like, you're headed for trouble. Especially if you start confiding in someone of the opposite sex.

Women Need To Make Sure Their Guys are Happy

The most successful swinging relationships I've seen are where the female half of the couple actively participates in finding women for her man to play with. I recognize that on the surface this sounds a little one-side, and it seems the male is the only one who would get any fun out of this arrangement.

Remember though, there are 2 to 3 times more single guys for a woman to play with than there are single females. When a female is too busy doing her own thing instead of making sure her guy has fun too, this can lead to a lot of frustration and resentment. One female I know will always make sure she goes out of her way to talk to the other females at the beginning of a party and let them know her man is interested. Some single females can be a little apprehensive about playing with guys who aren't single, so this is a good way to let them know they have the "greenlight" to be with your man. By doing this, she ensures that her man will have a good time while she's off having her own fun. Smart woman.

Beware of Hallpasses

A hallpass is when you let your partner go off and have sex with another person without you being around. When my wife and I would have a hallpass, we would make sure that it was on the same night for both of us, so one person wasn't just sitting around wondering what the other person was doing.

In hindsight, these hallpasses were probably not a good idea for us. Having one on one time with some of the opposite sex can lead to lots of different things that can be disastrous to your relationship.

Being alone with someone allows for the opportunity to become emotionally close to someone, and in most cases it's not a good idea.

It hurt our relationship, and we've also witnessed it destroy other marriages. You should also exercise extreme caution in allowing your partner to have a hallpass with a single person. I'm not trying to say that all hallpasses are evil, but just be extra careful and make sure that your relationship can handle it. After-sex cuddling and things like that should really be reserved for your spouse or partner in my opinion. If you're going to go through with a hallpass, it's very important that boundaries or rules are followed.

If you have a strict rule about kissing or oral sex, you should keep these same boundaries in place during your hallpass. Communication is always the key. Your partner is putting a tremendous amount of trust and faith in your hands by allowing you to have alone time with someone, so always remember that.

Chapter 5

Where To Find Other Swingers

So now you're ready to start swinging, but how do you find other like-minded couples?   This is probably a lot easier than you think.

Swinger Clubs

There are all kinds of swinger clubs in every state and in every major city, you just may not be aware of them.   A quick Google search is the best place to start looking.   Some swinger clubs are just "meet and greet" events where they may hold a gathering at a bar or some other establishment, and then any sexual activities would take place "off-premise" such as a hotel or someone's home. Depending on your location, there are also plenty of "on premise" clubs as well. These on premise clubs can make hooking up a little easier as most of them will have playrooms with beds and condoms.   In some of the more open-minded cities, the club may have a liquor license and dance floor to make mingling even easier. Sometimes clubs can be expensive as often they charge a membership fee, as well as an entry fee for that night.

There are two well-known swinger clubs in our area, so when we were first started out we did a tour of one. Most clubs will be more than happy to give you a tour of the place so you can decide if you wish to pursue a membership or not. The person who led us around was very friendly, and described all of the areas of the place as well as the rules. It did look a little run down, but it had two big hot tubs and porno playing on a huge TV screen. After our tour of the first place, my wife kind of felt like the place looked like a "flop house" (whore house) so we didn't purchase a membership. There also were a LOT of single males there that night, and we didn't see any single females. I thought it looked okay, but you know how we men are. We'll have sex on a cardboard box and not care. An important point here is always make sure both of you agree and feel comfortable before purchasing a membership.

A few months later we heard about a new club that opened up, and we decided to take a tour. The person who showed us around was friendly as well. She mentioned the club was in the process of getting its liquor license, which was a huge plus for us. She told us that a lot of people come just to watch and there is never any pressure to participate. We were also informed that on most nights they limit the number of single guys to 10, so that was a huge plus for me, plus they have security walking around at all times to make sure people are okay.

We really liked the fact that it had an upscale look to it, and they also had a couples lounge where only couples and single females are allowed.

We purchased a membership and a few weeks later finally got up the nerve to go back. We were both nervous as hell about going. We pulled into the parking garage and I actually thought about just turning around and going home. We took a deep breath and we went in, choosing to sit at the bar for a while. Looking back on that night, it's comical because we were so new to swinging, and we thought all we had to do was sit down and wait for people to proposition us. If you do choose to visit a swingers club, this is not the right attitude to have. Unless you two look like Brad Pitt and Angelina Jolie, people usually aren't going to be throwing themselves at you. Be sociable and say hello to a few people, and don't be afraid to strike up a conversation with someone.

What's even funnier is we sat at the bar for about an hour and no one spoke to us except for the occasional hello. As soon as I left to go to the bathroom and left my wife alone at the bar, this single guy tried to hit on her.   See, I told you that single guys get a bad rap in the swinger world, and rightfully so.

Later that night we found an empty bed in the couples lounge and started making out on it, and we eventually got naked. It was exciting watching all of the couples have sex, and knowing they were watching us as well. Upstairs there is an "orgy bar" with a really big bed, but it wasn't getting much action that night. There was one older single gentleman just walking around with his dick hanging out, like he was just waiting for some random woman to come up and grab it.   We decided to go back downstairs and had some more fun after we found an empty room. We left the door open so people could watch. Nothing like taking your wife doggy-style with a bunch of people watching. Later that night we also got to watch these two couples putting on a show in the same bed, and it ended with both guys having anal sex with the other guy's spouse. Both women squirted everywhere in orgasmic bliss. Damn that was great to watch.

One downside to these clubs is you can often see the same people over and over again. Because there aren't a ton of clubs, often once people find a place they enjoy they become lifelong visitors. On the one hand it's nice to feel like you're among friends, but if you're a new visitor it can almost make you feel like an outsider trying to join an established clique. No need to fear though, as almost everyone is warm and inviting to newcomers. Sometimes people like to avoid clubs because they fear running into someone they may know. This used to be a fear of ours too until we really thought about it. So what if we see someone we know? That person or couple is there for the same reason we are, so why should we be embarrassed? Just go with no expectations except to have fun, and you'll have an enjoyable time.

Swinging Websites

If you're not into the club scene, an easy way to get started is by joining a swingers website. There are numerous websites out there like adultfriendfinder.com, lovevoodoo.com, mixxxer.com, and many others. What's nice about these websites is you don't have to put up a picture of your face if you don't want to. What is also great is that most people will put up naked pictures of themselves, so you get so see right away what somebody is working with. This is a great way to meet other like-minded couples and singles without having to hang out in bars or clubs. You can browse profiles at your own leisure without any pressure, and you can send an e-mail to those you are interested in. If there is mutual interest, you can choose to meet at a place for drinks and/or dinner to see if you are compatible. What's good about this is you get a person or couple's undivided attention, instead of being at a club where so many people are fighting for attention.

One of the downsides though is that you often have to pay for a monthly membership to be able to contact anyone on the site. These monthly fees can be quite pricey with some charging almost $30 a month for membership. If you're a couple looking to meet a single guy, this is probably the easiest way to meet someone. Fortunately or unfortunately, websites are usually flooded with single guys. Beware though, some of these guys are married and just on there to cheat on their wives. If a guy is unwilling to trade face pictures with you, that's more than likely a dead give-away that he's a cheating spouse.

Another negative is this is one of the most difficult places to meet single women if you're looking for a threesome. I'd venture to guess that at least 30% of the single women profiles are fake. Some of the profiles are created by single guys trying to get revenge on their ex-girlfriends by posting nude pictures. What also happens is some females create profiles with no real intention of ever meeting anybody in person, as they just enjoy the ego boost from all the attention. We've also heard stories of some single guys posing as a couple, then when it's time to meet only a guy shows up, and he'll lie and say his wife couldn't come. If you're persistent and patient, you should find a few couples that you are compatible with. Often these couples are later able to point you to other couples they've had a good time with, and vice versa.

When setting up your profile, the more pictures the merrier. You'll find that couples with multiple pictures will get more action than those with just one or two. I also highly recommend cropping out any picture of your faces if you're nervous about anyone recognizing you. When you start communicating with other people, at that point you can send a picture of your faces if you desire. The great thing about not showing your face is it gives you the freedom to upload more provocative pictures.

More X-rated pictures equals more action. Nobody wants to see a picture of you posing with your pet dog, or some picture of you in a park looking at flowers. Remember that people will have hundreds of profiles to scroll through, so you need to catch their attention right away. I highly suggest that you have a sexy picture of your wife or girlfriend as your main profile picture. No offense guys but if a picture of your dick is your main picture, unless you're hung like an elephant nobody really cares. Now if it's a picture of your dick while you're receiving a blowjob or during sex, that's perfectly acceptable. The absolute BEST pictures to have on your profile will be of you having sex with another couple, woman, or male. This lets people know that you aren't flakes, and you're serious about meeting other like-minded people.

If you're looking at a single woman's profile, take a keen look at the number of pictures she has. If she's had an active profile for months and has only 2-3 face pictures on her profile, it's a good guess that the profile is probably fake. Even most "modest" women on the website will show a picture of their cleavage at least. Then there are the women on there who have tons of sexual pictures, but they're all solo pictures. Even if this isn't a fake profile, I'd venture to guess that this woman just enjoys all of the attention she gets and has no plan to ever meet anyone. She may even be married and on the website without her spouse's knowledge. I'm sure there are exceptions to this, but if a female is sexy and has lots of X-rated pictures of herself, you're telling me there's not at least ONE guy she could've taken a picture with while having sex? Sounds fishy to me. Of course some women will feign interest in meeting, only to cancel on you at the last minute. Some of the excuses we've heard are:

"My cat got sick"

"We just bought our Christmas tree, and we HAVE to put it up tonight"

"My ex borrowed my car and hasn't come back with it"

In my single days, there was nothing worse than seeing an attractive woman online, going to meet her and she shows up looking like one of the creatures from Lord of The Rings. Unfortunately this happens on swinger websites as well. The very first person we met from one of these websites was a single guy. I remember looking at this guy's pictures, and even I was envious of how he looked. The guy had a build like Dwayne "The Rock" Johnson and six-pack abs. His profile said he was in his 40's. Hell, I would've been honored for him to have sex with my wife. The guy who showed up though was at LEAST in his mid-fifties and I'm pretty certain I was in better shape than he was. We were polite though and had a conversation with him for a few hours before parting. In hindsight, we should have gotten up and left as soon as he sat down. Unfortunately this type of thing is very common on both regular dating websites and swinger websites. Don't feel like you have to sit there and put up with someone who was dishonest about their looks, and you aren't being rude by calling them out on it.

Swinger Resorts

Swinger Resorts, in my opinion, are some of the BEST places to meet like-minded adults while having a ton of fun. What can be better by going to a place where all of the alcohol is included in the price, plus you're surrounded by naked people having fun?

People thought we were crazy when we said we were getting married at a clothing-optional resort. It was our first time visiting a nude resort, and we were both nervous and excited. We weren't swingers at the time, and my wife thought there would be all kinds of naked people trying to have sex with us, so she almost backed out a few times. We chose Desire Resorts in Mexico since it was a couples-only resort. This was also our first time at an all-inclusive resort. There's nothing like waking up with a mimosa, then floating around a pool all day drinking alcohol.

For the first two days, I kept my swim trunks on and my wife kept on her swimsuit. By day three I was naked, and my wife was topless. By day five we were both walking around naked. One of the things I feared as man was getting an erection in public, but that never happened. Then of course you think everyone will be looking at you, and you'll feel out of place. On the contrary, we actually felt more self-conscious with our clothes on than without.   The great thing about clothing-optional resorts is there are all shapes and sizes with no one being judgmental.

Of course my wife's fears were never realized, and no one was aggressive at all.   Everyone was so nice and friendly towards us, and even did shots with us when we told them we were getting married on the beach.   One of the couples was even nice enough to get dressed up and attend our wedding ceremony.   This vacation completely blew our misconception about swingers out of the water.   I loved how friendly and open everyone was.   You could be naked in the pool with a doctor, a waitress, or an engineer and no one cares.   Everyone just has a great time, and in my opinion everyone being nude encourages people to be more social. If you're a couple and looking for your first clothing-optional resort, Desire Resorts in Mexico is a great place to choose because it's couples-only.

Our second clothing-optional trip was at the world famous Hedonism II in Jamaica. We'd never been to Jamaica before, and by this trip we had discussed swinging and felt like we were ready for it.   Needless to say we were really looking forward to the trip. To be fair, most of Hedonism's rooms are very outdated, but as of this writing I've heard there is a major renovation going on, and all the rooms are getting updated. Honestly though, you're only going to be in your room to sleep and have sex.

The resort has a clothing side, and a nude side. Once again, people of all shapes, sizes, and races were represented so there is never a need to feel self-conscious. If you think you're too big to be walking around nude, just trust me you'll run across somebody who will be way bigger. Plus with all the free alcohol flowing, nobody cares anyway. There was this one woman who easily weighed over 300 lbs out there strutting her stuff, and all the Jamaican men loved her. Hedonism II has a reputation for being wild and freaky, and this can vary depending on when you're there. You'll see all types of people there, as we even sat in the nude pool one afternoon with a certain Texas politician.

We went to the nude pool for the first time, and I think we had this idea that people would just be groping each other and having sex all over the place, but it wasn't like that at all. Like I've said before, swingers are some of the nicest people you will ever run across. How can you be mean if you're willing to be naked around complete strangers. One thing about Hedonism II that is different is they do allow single people to attend. Once again, because we were new to swinging we had this misconception that we would just sit back, and everyone would want to fuck us. So we were a little bewildered when no one was approaching us at all. We talked with one of the other couples about this, and they laughed. They said that since we were pretty much clinging to each other all the time and not really talking to others, most people just assumed we weren't swingers and didn't want to be bothered. So in other words since we weren't being outwardly friendly, we weren't really giving off the "swinger vibe".

It was a little strange for us because swinging can be like learning how to date all over again. How do I approach someone I'm interested in? How do I know if they want to have sex or not? Then to compound the fact, we were worried that the other one of us would get mad if we started talking to somebody we were attracted to. See why open communication is so important? Soon we opened up and started talking to more people in the nude pool. I remember we were talking to this one couple from New York, and the guy's wife started stroking my dick under the water. After the couple left, I was faced with a dilemma. Do I tell my wife about it and risk her getting mad, or do I just keep it to myself? Since we were so new to it all, we didn't really know how to react in these types of situations. I ended up telling my wife about it, and she was fine with it.

What's funny though is later that week, I was going to the pool bar to get a drink and I started chatting with this woman. My dick started getting hard because the woman was rubbing up against me, so I had to wait a while before walking out of the pool to go over to the hot tub area. My wife wasn't too happy with "some ugly woman" being able to give me an erection. Why do women think that our dicks are connected to an on/off switch and we turn off our erections on cue? Anyway, that's another topic for another day....

Remember that couple from New York where the wife was stroking my dick under the water? Later on that week we decided to hook up with them and got our swingers cherry popped so to speak. We also hooked up with another single male while were there, and gave my wife a threesome. If you do decide to visit Hedonism II, here are some tips for a great time:

1. Guys, carry condoms at ALL times. Even if you're in the nude pool completely naked, put some condoms in your towel or something. You NEVER know when a female will want to hook up, and the last thing you want is to not have any condoms handy.

2. Get a room on the nude side. Most of the fun happens on the nude side. Also if you're looking to hook up, you don't want to drag your willing fuck buddy (or buddies) all the way back to the other side of the resort to get to your room. You know how fickle some women can be. If they want to have sex, they want it NOW, not 15 minutes from now. Yes the nude side is more expensive, but it's worth it since that's where everybody hangs out.

3. Stay up late. A lot of the naughty action takes place after midnight in the nude pool, which we seemed to keep missing since we weren't staying up late. One night a woman was on a table in the pool and people would spin her around. Whoever her pussy landed in front of went down on her. Fun times. I would suggest taking a nap during the middle of the day so you'll have more energy at night.

4. Ladies, if one of the locals asks if you want some "Jamaican Lobster", they mean dick. Be careful about going somewhere off the resort with a stranger because they may not drop you back off at the resort. This happened to a

woman, and she ended up having to walk a few miles back to the resort.

5. I know I sound like a broken record, but if you're a couple you need to discuss what is and isn't okay before you go. We should've done this, and we would've had way more fun if we weren't wondering if it was okay to approach somebody. For people who are new to swinging, Hedonism II is another great place to get started because everybody is so friendly and approachable. Also, you never have to see any of the people again in case you're worried about your spouse becoming attached to someone.

6. Watch the alcohol intake your first day. When we arrived, we immediately started drinking by the pool. The combination of all that alcohol, the heat, and humidity can really do a number on you. That next day my wife spent the entire day in bed trying to recover. One of the bartenders told us that this happens quite often to visitors on their first day.

7. If you want marijuana, just ask somebody on the staff. For the first two days we kept smelling weed all around the pool but never saw any. Finally one day we were waiting in line

for breakfast, and a chef asked us if we had everything we needed. We said yes, but then he asked again if we REALLY had everything we needed. My wife goes, "Well, we've been smelling some stuff in the air, but we don't know where to get any.". Chef tells us to come back in about 20 minutes. We show up, and he points us over to some guy. On the beach you will find all kinds of vendors selling pipes and rolling paper.

There are lots of other great resorts out there too like Caliente Caribe in the Dominican Republic, Garden of Eden Resort in Panama, and Spice Lanzarote in Spain. Like I stated at the beginning of this book, there are also nude cruises you can go on. What's better than seeing the world, being naked, and meeting some awesome people?

Chapter 6

Throwing a Swingers Party

So you've been swinging for a while and you enjoy it. At some point you may get tired of going to the swinger clubs, and you may feel like hosting your own swingers party. My wife and I did this after we got tired of seeing the same people all the time at the swingers club we frequent. One thing that is great about house parties is because they are smaller in nature, people usually will open up and talk more to each other since it's a more intimate setting. Here are a few tips I've gathered on how to throw a great party.

Don't Be Afraid to Ask People to Contribute

Don't feel awkward or weird about asking people to contribute in some way to the party. Look at it this way. The swingers club we visit charges an entry fee of $40-$60 for a couple, and that doesn't even include purchasing a membership if you aren't a member.

Then throw in the cost of drinks. Let's say a 3 month membership costs you $40. So it's not out of the realm to say a couple could easily spend over $100 going to a swingers club.

At our parties, we would ask people to bring a bottle of their favorite alcohol to share to add to our existing alcohol, and we would cook up a bunch of finger food and appetizers. Your guests will spend a lot less money bringing a bottle of alcohol than they would at a swingers club. Also, it's been our experience that you are more likely to get laid at a house party than you will at a club. We know of another couple that will throw parties at a hotel suite and will usually ask couples to pay a $10 entry fee.

Condoms, Clean Sheets, and Towels

Don't forget to put a bowl of condoms in each room, as you want to encourage people to have safe sex, and you don't want your guests stumbling around trying to find a condom during the heat of the moment. You will also want to provide a change of bedsheets in each room, as well as towels. Don't worry about buying expensive sheets, the cheap sheets will work fine. Also you may want to invest in some air mattresses to give your guests more options for fun. I would also suggest buying some waterproof mattress protectors as well. You can easily buy an assorted pack of 100 condoms on Amazon or from adameve.com for cheap. If someone is allergic to latex or only uses a certain brand of condom, they can feel free to bring their own condoms.

Guys, you may also want to order some "little blue pills" before the big event because there's a good possibility of you having sex multiple times that night.   You may be laughing right now, but I can promise you that you won't be laughing if you're at a party and you start having performance anxiety.   It can happen to anyone, and of course the more you focus on trying to get an erection, the worse it will become.   Worse yet, the female you're with may not be willing to give you a second chance since there are plenty of other males around.

I remember one night we invited this couple over, and the husband and I were both having some "difficulties" performing. That was not a fun night by any means, so spare yourself the trouble before something like that happens. My "go to" website is bmpharmacy.com for ordering pills. They even have liquid packs that you can carry in your pocket, and they start working a lot faster than the pills do. Better to be safe than sorry. My party routine is to masturbate earlier that evening before the party, then later take a pill or a shot of liquid right when the party starts. For me this helps to prevent any premature ejaculation issues that might happen, and I usually will have a lot more stamina than usual. Remember that the swinger community in your area really isn't that big, and everyone tends to know each other through mutual associations. Females talk, and you don't want to be known for ejaculating too quickly or being unable to perform. My technique may not work for you, so you may want to experiment with a few different things that may be more suitable for you.

Meet People Before Inviting Them

I strongly suggest meeting people before inviting them, especially if you are going to have the party at your house. Some people will post the details of their party on a swinger website, and that's fine if that works for you. We always liked to be in control of who was going to show up. This one hotel party we went to, some of the guys just seemed to be "weirdos" and we didn't really like the vibe. We felt like having more control over the people we invited made for a better party. Also as the man of the house, you may want to walk around and check out all of the action that's going on. If you see a female looking around like she needs help if some guy has her cornered, you will want to step in and help out. You always want to make sure your single female guests feel safe if they come alone.

There was this one single guy at our party who ended up calling a female a stuck up bitch because she didn't want to have sex with him. We immediately made him leave our party and he's never been invited back. Another time, this overly aggressive guy smacked a female's ass so hard that she got upset. This guy really made a poor judgement call as he didn't ask for permission before doing so, and the woman's boyfriend got really upset as well. This same guy later just started kissing on one of the wives without asking for permission and the female pushed him away. Needless to say he hasn't been invited to another party either.

Make Most of the Males Bring a Female Date

When we first started swinging, we were having a hard time meeting females. One of the things I did was to find some single males to invite to our party, but I required them to bring a female.

This serves a few purposes. For one, it keeps your party from becoming a sausage fest.

(Trust me, at LEAST two of the females who accept your invite will flake out and not show up) Also, we find that males who can bring a date are usually little better behaved. Third, this is a GREAT way to meet more single females. My first threesome came about this way, because I got the phone number from one of the females who was brought along as a date, and we set up a threesome a few weeks later. A lot of single guys will try and act like they don't have anyone to bring and will try to come solo, but don't allow this. Trust me, those single guys know at least one freaky female they can invite. One guy was awesome enough to show up with two females at one of our parties.

Invite the Freakiest Female You Know

The first time you throw a party and get a group of people together, everyone will be a little nervous and anxious. It's like everyone is standing around...making conversation...but everyone's scared to make that first move, or be the first one to get naked. Enter your freaky friend.

See, the freaky female friend serves multiple purposes. By freaky I mean a female who loves to have sex and won't hesitate to get naked. At for our first party, we were 2 hours in and everyone was still talking, no one had taken the plunge yet. Finally 30 more minutes went by, one of our female friends went and changed clothes. She came out wearing just a robe, pulled out a dildo, got on our couch and started pleasing herself with the dildo. After about 5 minutes of watching, a guy walked over to her and they started having fun. Then everybody loosened up and people started rubbing and feeling on each other.

Having a freaky female friend helps get the party started, and because she loves to have sex she will make sure all the guys (and females in this case, since our friend is bi-sexual) at your party have a great time. Remember, as a male the last thing you want is to be competing for women at your own party.

Don't Invite "Miss Too Good" for Everyone

Everyone has a female friend like this.   She's attractive, but she thinks she looks better than she actually does.   You would think that having an attractive female like this would be ideal for your sex party, but nothing could be further from the truth.   Because she is likely to be so picky, she will probably spend most of her time pointing out the physical flaws of all the guys at your party, which in turn can influence some of the other women to start thinking they shouldn't be having sex with those guys either.

This sounds childish, but peer pressure like this can kill the vibe of a party quickly.   A woman may see a guy and think he's sort of cute and might be thinking of hooking up with him that night.   Then your friend says something like "He looks okay but he's too chubby. No way would I want to see him naked."   Now the woman is second-guessing herself, and now she's thinking that she doesn't want to hook up with someone who's "below the standards" of this other woman.

This peer pressure will also influence other guys as well.   I've seen jealousy rear its ugly head at some of our parties, and certain women may not like the fact that one woman in particular is getting all the action.   I overheard a woman telling some of the guys that she didn't think one of the women was pretty at all, and she couldn't understand why everybody wanted to hook up with her. She also said there's no way she could sleep with a guy who wanted to be with this "unattractive" female. As a result, some of the guys who wanted to hook up with her didn't do so, because they didn't want to mess up their chance of getting some action from "Miss Too Good For Everybody". The sad part of this is that "Miss Too Good For Everybody" often spends the majority of her time talking down about everybody else instead of enjoying herself. To make matters worse, if this type of woman is your girlfriend or spouse, you'll never truly be able to enjoy yourself at a party because you're too worried about finding women that meets her stamp of approval.

Account For the Flakes

Always have a contingency plan for the people who are going to flake. The people most likely to flake on your party will be the females. As stated earlier, you should expect at least two of the females you invite to stand you up. You'll need to start recognizing the ones who are most likely to flake on you. The keywords for a flake are "maybe", "I think so", or "I'll have to see". Any person who says this will probably be a flake, and you might as well plan on them not showing up. We would always invite around 25 people, knowing that only 15 or so would actually show up. Don't get too disheartened by the no shows and flakes. I personally think there is zero excuse for just not showing up. At least be an adult and let someone know you don't plan to attend. Sometimes people are good at wasting other people's time, and that's a shame. Time is the one commodity you can never get back, and people who flake on you obviously don't value your time.

Expect The Unexpected, and Don't Get Frustrated

If you're throwing your party with your partner or spouse, you two need to discuss any rules you two have prior to the party. Always know though, sometimes things will not go as planned. The first party we hosted was close to my birthday, so the plan was for my wife to round up at least two other women for me and then go upstairs to have a foursome with me.

Like I said, that was the plan. What ended up happening is one of the guys took my half-drunk wife by the hand into our bedroom and I didn't see much of her until the party was pretty much over, except for me checking on her from time to time to make sure she was okay. Every time she finished with one guy, another guy would be coming into our bedroom so she was "hosting" in her own special way.

Finally near the end of the night, I got frustrated and went to find some women of my own. I let them know what was supposed to happen for my birthday, and two women agreed to go upstairs with me.   As a tangent, a key point here to keep in mind is that with swinging (and in life in general I think) you are responsible for our own happiness. Don't sit back and wait for someone else to make something happen for you, just go do it yourself.

So the two women were on me for all of about 3 minutes, and then 2 guys came in and started playing with the women. The one that was giving me a blowjob at the time started getting penetrated from behind, so she lost her concentration so to speak and forgot about me. Then two more people came into the room, so there was a total of about six people all on the bed and I was at the bottom of the pile, mad as hell that my first attempt at a threesome was ruined. (Note to the other men reading this. If you're at a party and you're about to get a threesome, lock the door so other guys don't ruin it.)

There was also another point at that same party where I was sitting on the couch with a woman, and she told me to go get a condom. I ran upstairs to get a condom, sat back down on the couch and put the condom on. Well at that particular moment she walked outside with her husband to smoke a cigarette. So there I sat on the couch with a hard dick wearing a condom while they smoked. Talk about a frustrating night.

There was another party we attended where all hell broke loose. One of the single guys was having sex with someone's drunk wife and wasn't wearing a condom. The husband saw this, and the woman had to keep her husband from going to get his gun. To make it worse, the guy was someone the wife invited without her husband knowing about it. Needless to say this guy was kicked out of the party, and the whole vibe was ruined.

Just remember, something will probably happen during the course of the night that you have no control over, or something won't go as planned and you'll become frustrated.

Conclusion

So I hope by now you've got a good idea of how to get started in the swinging lifestyle. Like I've stated often throughout this guide, communication with your partner is the number one thing that will make for an enjoyable time as you begin your journey. Hopefully I've given you both the great and not-so-great aspects of swinging.

If you have any questions, comments or concerns, you can feel free to contact me at swingersguru@gmail.com and I'll try my best to answer. If you enjoyed my book, it would consider it an honor if you'd be willing to give my book a good review. You can also check out my blog at andrekeith.blogspot.com. Here are some of the most common questions I've been asked:

Q: How Do I Convince My Partner to Start Swinging?

A: This answer is a little tricky. The first thing I would ask is what kind of person is your partner? If your partner is possessive, insecure, and has jealousy issues you have no business at all wanting to introduce swinging into your relationship. If you're with someone that gets upset if you even look in the direction of another person, or if your relationship is already in trouble, then swinging is not right for you at all. Remember if you already have problems in your relationship, swinging will just make them worse.

Now with that being said, if you have a good relationship there are a few ways you can bring up the topic of swinging. I think one of the best ways to start this conversation is after a good night of sex with your partner. As with anything you are trying to sell, (you're trying to sell your partner on the idea) you always have to make the other person knows what's in it for them. If your partner is undecided, you really aren't going to get anywhere if you keep talking about what's in it for you.

During the afterglow of sex, why not ask your partner what kind of fantasies they have. Ladies, ask your guy if he's ever had a fantasy of being with two women at the same time. Guys, you can always ask your partner if she's ever had any fantasies of being with another woman, or with two guys at the same time. Even during sex, you can sometimes have a night of dirty talk with your partner and talk about different scenarios like other people watching, or even joining in. If this turns your partner on, this could be a sign that your partner may be open to some of those fantasies becoming a reality.

I have to caution you though that just because someone has a fantasy, it doesn't always mean they want it to happen. Sometimes fantasies are better left in the imagination. If your partner isn't interested in the swinger lifestyle at all, you will just have to accept that and respect your partner's wishes.

Q: What was it like watching your wife have sex with another guy?

A: I'm going to be completely honest here, it was very weird. The first time it happened for us was at Hedonism II. It was almost like an out of body experience, where I really couldn't believe I was watching this happen. It was kind of strange for my wife as well, and she said she really couldn't get into it like she thought she could. The first time you do anything that pushes you out of your comfort zone will always feel a little strange and awkward. I know this answer surprises some of you, but I don't believe in feeding people a bunch of BS when it comes to giving honest answers about swinging.

Q: What happens if someone becomes attached to my partner?

A: Sometimes this does happen unfortunately. It could be a single female, single male, or even someone from a couple who becomes too attached.   All of a sudden you will start to get this weird dislike for a particular person, and you can't quite place your finger on it. I think the most effective way to deal with this is to take a break from being around this person, or cut this person completely off. You and your partner should have an agreement that at any point if you say that someone is off-limits, then you both should abide by that rule.   I am a firm believer in trusting your gut instincts about someone when it comes to swinging.

One of the best ways to avoid this is for guys to communicate with the guys, and for women to communicate with women.   For clarification, this means that if you meet another couple and you get along great, the guys should exchange numbers with each other, and the females should do the same.   This serves as a great way to keep boundaries in place, and it's especially important for dealing with single females and single males.   If after a certain amount of time you feel comfortable enough, you can then let your partner communicate with this other person.

Remember, swinging is supposed to be fun and exciting, and it shouldn't be causing you any additional stress or anxiety.

Q: Is there ever any jealousy among swingers?

A: Yes.   People who love each other will experience jealousy from time to time, but this isn't necessarily a bad thing.   A little jealousy in a relationship is actually healthy.   Jealousy in a relationship is like putting salt in food.   A little bit enhances things, but too much will completely ruin everything.   Most couples we've talked to who are honest will admit to having a little jealousy from time to time.   It could be that you don't like the way your partner was passionately kissing someone after sex, or you got jealous because your partner was moaning louder with someone else than they ever have with you.

The most important thing here once again is communication.   If you're feeling this way after a night of swinging, talk about it with your partner. The absolute worst thing you can do is to hold in your feelings of jealousy or resentment because it will end up coming out in a way you don't expect.   We're only human, and because no one is perfect you will eventually do something while swinging that your partner won't like.

Q: How do we find a female for a threesome?

A: Guys, here is a question you need to ask yourselves. If your woman wanted a threesome with another man, would you give her one? If your answer is no, then you have no business asking your wife to give you one. What's fair is fair. Now if you answered yes or your wife has no desire to be with another man, then please proceed.

This one can be a little tricky. The most obvious way is to get on a swingers website, and search for single females. Remember though, pretty much every single male and every other couple is looking for the same thing, so there will be lots of competition. Also keep in mind that probably 30% of the single females will have a fake profile. Then throw in the fact that another 20% will be flakes and have no intention of ever meeting anyone. You can see now how it would be difficult to catch a single female's attention on a swingers website. If this is the avenue you choose in your quest for a threesome, there is only one way to stand out from the competition.

Be in shape, and be sexy.

I know most of you won't like that answer, but it's the cold hard truth. Why would a sexy female who has literally hundreds of people trying to get her attention be drawn to an out-of-shape couple? Yes I know, you and your wife have wonderful personalities and you give regularly to charity. Swinging is about sex and raw animal instinct. You could be the greatest two people in the world but no one cares because they only thing people really care about on a website is how you look. As a matter of fact, if your pictures aren't attractive and sexy no one is even going to bother with reading what your profile says. Harsh, but it's the truth.

One of the best ways to get a threesome in my opinion, is to start getting to know more of the couples. Once you've found a few couples that you enjoy having sex with, they may know a few single females that you may be interested in. If you two are great in bed and are respectful, the other couple will have no problem introducing you to some of their female friends. Even better yet if the husband trusts you enough, he may be willing to let his wife have a hallpass with you guys if you're willing to return the favor.

Also, I suggested earlier in the book that if you throw your own swingers party, be sure to invite a few single males but require them to bring a female date. We spent almost an entire year looking for a female on a swingers website with no luck. After we hosted our first swingers party, I had my threesome within 3 weeks. As an added bonus, since private parties are smaller in nature, this is a chance where you can truly let your personality shine in your favor and win people over. If you become known for throwing great parties where you make sure your guests have fun and you make the single women feel safe, you'll have lots of threesomes lined up in no time at all.

The one thing that's tricky about threesomes with a female is you need to let your lady take the lead in this department. If you're at a party or club, often things will go a lot faster if your woman takes the initiative and starts talking to some of the other women. Remember, a lot of single females don't want to approach a man who's part of a couple for fear of upsetting the wife. Also, this allows your lady to choose another female that SHE thinks is attractive and is also comfortable with.

If you as a male walk over and starts talking to her, you can bet that she may feel a little uneasy and may keep glancing at your wife/girlfriend to see if she's getting upset. One of our single female friends says that she always worries about playing with a couple, because she doesn't want the wife to think she's trying to steal her husband. If your wife walks over and lets it be known that you both find her sexy, then most of the apprehension goes out of the door.

As a side note about threesomes, be sure not to waste too much time on people that are flakes, or fixating on just one female. If you search the swinger websites long enough, you will eventually find a female who seems like she's interested.   Or you may meet a female from a party who claims to be interested in participating in a threesome. If you make a few attempts at trying to arrange a meeting with this woman and she always has an excuse, it's best to just ignore her and keep looking for other prospects.

Even female friends that you already know may think they're interested in giving you a threesome, but when it comes down to it they're too scared to take any action. I can't tell you how many females over the years have said they would have a threesome with us, but there was always an excuse or some other lame reason.

Always remember that in life, if someone truly wants to accomplish something, they'll figure out a way to make it happen. Before our first FMF threesome, we had a female friend of ours who would promise all the time that she wanted a threesome with us. Months and months of waiting, and the threesome never happened.

When we had our first threesome with a single female, we set a date for it to happen, and she came over that night. No bullshit, no one million questions, no lame excuses. Your time is way too valuable to waste on people who are full of excuses, so I always suggest to stop wasting your time with these people, because the only thing it will lead to is frustration.

Q: How do we arrange a threesome with another guy?

A: This one is super easy. Go onto any swingers website and put in your profile that you are looking for a single guy. I can promise you it will take less than a day for you to get at least 15 emails. The upside to having so many guys to choose from is it allows you to be very picky. Take your time and read through the profiles together carefully. Always feel free to ask the guy for a picture of his face before meeting. If he objects with some excuse, or says he has to be very discreet and you can see his face in person, then I would move on because the guy is probably married or in a relationship.

No matter how careful you are though, you can still be fooled. We met this one guy we both thought was pretty cool, and we eventually thought of him as a friend. He started getting a little too clingy at one point so we cut him loose. Later we found out that he had been in a long-term relationship that whole time, obviously hooking up with other people without his girlfriend's knowledge.

www.ingramcontent.com/pod-product-compliance
Lightning Source LLC
Chambersburg PA
CBHW070807290526
45795CB00002B/648